Excursion Inside:

Unwinding the Riddle of Disease Cells

By

Racheal B. Ajose

Table of Contents

Introduction   5
Part 2:   7
Transformation and Metamorphosis   7
Part 3:   8
Infinitesimal Battlefield   8
Part 4:   9
Attack and Metastasis   9
Part 5:   10
Progressive Therapies   10
Part 6:   11
Voices of Resilience   11
Part 7:   12
Moral Quandaries and Future Frontiers   12
Part 8:   13
Exposing Cell Mysteries   13
Part 9:   14
From Seat to Bedside: Translational Medicine   14
Part 10:   15
Worldwide Viewpoints on Malignant Growth Difficulties and Collaborations   15
Part 11:   16
Craftsmanship and Science Impact: The Visual Story of Disease Cells   16
Part 12:   17
Past the Cells: Effect on Society and Culture   17
Part 13:   18
Unknown Regions: Investigating Rising Frontiers   18
   19
Part 14:   19
Exploring Vulnerability: The Human Experience of Cancer   19
Part 15:   20
Past Limits: Worldwide Joint Efforts in Disease Research   20
Part 16:   21
What was to come Disclosed: Patterns and Prospects in Disease Research   21
Part 17:   22
Moral Outskirts in Malignant Growth Exploration and Treatment   22
Part 18:   23
The Interconnected Web: Social and Ecological Effects on Cancer   23
Part 19:   24
The Force of Avoidance: Techniques and Innovations   24
Part 20:   25
Reflections and Future Horizons   25
Part 21:   26

Connecting Disciplines: The Union of Oncology and Technology   26

Part 22:   27

The Human Touch in Oncology: Sympathy, Correspondence, and Palliative Care   27

Part 23:   28

Worldwide Backing and Strategy: Molding the Oncology Landscape   28

Part 24:   29

The Strength of the Human Soul: Accounts of Win and Hope   29

Part 25:   30

Reflections on the Excursion: An Embroidery of Understanding   30

Index: 31

Assets and Further Reading   31

Introduction

In the mind-boggling embroidery of life, a troublesome power arises at the cell level—the beginning of defiance. Welcome to "Excursion Inside: Disentangling the Puzzle of Malignant Growth Cells." In this investigation, we set out on a spellbinding odyssey into the tiny world, where the narrative of disease cells unfolds.

A Minute Odyssey Begins

The excursion starts with the introduction of malignant growth cells, as we disentangle the secrets encompassing their beginning. From the perplexing dance of hereditary qualities to the outside sets off that set up for disobedience, we dig into the starting points of this imposing enemy.

The Concealed Battles

As we explore the minuscule war zone, witness the steady battle between the safe framework and disease cells. Find out how science is reshaping this milestone, with notable immunotherapies offering new expectations and conceivable outcomes.

Transformation and Invasion

Our investigation reaches out to the changes and transformations that characterize disease cells. Follow their risky excursion as they attack encompassing tissues and set out on the overwhelming journey for far-off organs—the actual embodiment of metastasis.

Reforming the Fight

In the midst of the difficulties, progressive treatments arise. From designated therapies to the commitment of customized medication, we witness the development of disease care and the reshaping of survival potential.

Voices that Reverberate Resilience

Entwined inside the logically embroidered artwork are the voices of flexibility—individual stories of wins, challenges, and the significant effect of logical progressions. These accounts help us to remember the human soul's perseverance through strength, even with difficulty.

Morals and Future Frontiers

Mull over the moral difficulties presented by arising advances in disease research. Look into the future boondocks of accurate medication and customized treatments, exploring the fragile harmony between advancement and moral contemplations.

As we leave on this "Excursion Inside," get ready to unwind the intricacies of malignant growth cells, from their beginning to the very front of logical leaps forward. This book is a challenge to investigate, comprehend, and value the determined quest for information in the continuous fight against perhaps humankind's most imposing enemy.

In the initial part, "Beginning of Resistance," we set out on an excursion to uncover the strange starting points of disease cells. The account dives into the complexities of their starting point, investigating the cell occasions and ecological elements that trigger the beginning of uncontrolled development.

1.1 The Introduction of Malignant Growth Cells

Investigate how ordinary cell processes turned out badly, prompting the arrangement of disease cells. Explore the job of hereditary transformations and their effect on cell conduct.

Triggers and Initiators
Inspect outer factors like natural openings, way of life decisions, and hereditary inclinations that act as triggers for the resistance inside cells.
Comprehend how a blend of components can make way for the improvement of harmful cells.

Unwinding the Secrets of Oncogenesis
Reveal the mind-boggling components engaged with oncogenesis, the cycle by which typical cells change into malignant growth cells.
Feature key achievements in logical comprehension that have unwound the secrets of the beginning of resistance at the cell level.

"Beginning of Disobedience" sets the stage for the investigation of disease cells, offering bits of knowledge into the crucial points in time and factors that start their degenerate way inside the human body.

Part 2:

Transformation and Metamorphosis

In this part, we dive into the perplexing universe of hereditary changes and the transformation that characterizes the existence pattern of malignant growth cells. From the inconspicuous changes inside the cell code to the significant effect on conduct, we disentangle the hereditary embroidery that moves cells on a path of uncontrolled development.

2.1 The Hereditary Embroidered Artwork of Cancer

Investigate the assorted cluster of hereditary changes that can drive the change of typical cells into dangerous substances.
Grasp the job of changes in modifying cell work and advancing unrestrained multiplication.

2.2 Variation and Evolution

Dive into the versatile idea of disease cells, analyzing how they develop to conquer hindrances and lodge the body's protection systems.
Reveal the procedures utilized by malignant growth cells to flourish in different microenvironments.

2.3 Hereditary Transformations: Impetuses of Change

Explore explicit hereditary changes that assume critical roles in the movement of different diseases.
Inspect the powerful interaction between hereditary changes and the cell microenvironment, molding the course of transformation.

As we venture through the intricacies of transformation, a more profound comprehension of the sub-atomic complexities driving malignant growth's movement will emerge. This section fills in as a passage to the versatile scene where the hereditary code goes through significant changes, making way for the steady quest for endurance by malignant growth cells.

Part 3:

Infinitesimal Battlefield

Step onto the war zone, inconspicuous to the unaided eye, where the resistant framework compensate
for a determined conflict against disease cells. In this part, we enlighten the minuscule battles,
uncovering the multifaceted dance between the body's protectors and the defiant powers of disease.

3.1 The Safe Framework's Defense

Reveal the complexities of how the safe framework distinguishes and targets malignant growth cells
as strange substances.
Investigate the job of safe cells, like immune system microorganisms and normal executioner cells, in
the reconnaissance and end of dangerous dangers.

3.2 Immunotherapies: Another Frontier

Venture through the state-of-the art domain of immunotherapies, finding how these therapies saddle
the force of a safe framework to battle disease.
Investigate the commitment and difficulties of designated spot inhibitors, vehicle lymphocyte
treatment, and other inventive immunotherapeutic methodologies.

3.3 Tackling the Force of the Insusceptible System

Dive into the developing scene of customized immunotherapies, fitting medicines to the individual's
safe profile.
Look at the forward leaps that mark a change in perspective in disease treatment, underscoring the
harmonious connection between science and the body's normal safeguards.

In the minuscule combat zone, where cells conflict and safe sentinels stand monitor, this section
reveals insight into the unique cooperations molding the course of the conflict against malignant
growth. From the cutting edges of logical development to the capability of customized resistance-
based treatments, we witness the continuous battle to influence the situation for mending and strength

Part 4:

Attack and Metastasis

Set out on an excursion through the unsafe scene of intrusion and metastasis, where malignant growth cells leave on an extraordinary odyssey, exploring tissues and chasing after far-off organs. In this part, we unwind the components and secrets behind the spread of disease, uncovering the significant difficulties presented by metastatic excursions.

4.1 The Unsafe Excursion Begins
Investigate the underlying strides of intrusion as disease cells split away from their starting point and penetrate tissues close by.
Comprehend the signs and variations that empower malignant growth cells to start the excursion towards metastasis.

4.2 Exploring Tissues and Organs
Follow the metastatic path as malignant growth cells explore through the circulation system or lymphatic framework, looking for new regions.
Analyze the cooperation between coursing growth cells and the microenvironments of far-off organs.

4.3 Metastasis Disclosed: Experiences into Spread
Disclose the complexities of metastasis, from the arrangement of auxiliary growths to the difficulties presented by the host climate.
Investigate the effect of metastasis on treatment procedures and the journey for helpful intercessions to stop or hinder this impressive cycle.

In the domain of intrusion and metastasis, this section reveals insight into the exceptional flexibility of disease cells, their excursion through the body, and the logical undertakings pointed toward understanding and controlling their steady quest for new regions.

Part 5:

Progressive Therapies

In this section, we explore the scene of progressive treatments that are reshaping the account of disease care. From designated accuracy therapies to the commitment of customized medication, witness the development of helpful methodologies that hold the possibility to rethink the results of the fight against disease.

5.1 Designated Treatments: Accuracy in Action

Investigate the accuracy of designated treatments intended to explicitly disturb the sub-atomic systems driving disease cell development.
Analyze how recognizing and focusing on unambiguous atoms can prompt more powerful and less harmful treatment methodologies.

5.2 Customized Medication: Fitting Treatments

Uncover the idea of customized medication, where medicines are custom-made to the interesting hereditary and sub-atomic profiles of individual patients.
Investigate the effect of genomic and sub-atomic profiling in directing treatment choices and working on restorative results.

5.3 Leap Forward: Changing Malignant Growth Care

Venture through the leaps forward that are changing the scene of malignant growth care, from immunotherapies to quality treatments.
Comprehend how these original methodologies are offering new expectations and further developing endurance rates for patients confronting different types of disease.

In the domain of progressive treatments, this section enlightens the steps made in accuracy and customized medication, displaying the force of advancement in the persistent quest for compelling and designated therapies for people wrestling with the intricacies of disease.

Part 6:

Voices of Resilience

In this part, we enhance the human side of the disease story, delivering the voices of versatility—individual accounts of wins, challenges, and the significant effect of logical headways on the existences of those impacted.

6.1 Individual Stories of Triumph
Hear the motivating accounts of people who have confronted the impressive difficulties of disease with fortitude and strength.
Investigate the victories that go beyond the clinical domain, mirroring the strength of the human soul notwithstanding misfortune.

6.2 Difficulties and Wins Along the Journey
Explore the high points and low points of the disease venture, recognizing the difficulties faced by patients, guardians, and their encouraging groups of people.
Feature the snapshots of flexibility and assurance that arise in the midst of the intricacies of determination, treatment, and recuperation.

6.3 The Human Side of Disease Research
Acquire bits of knowledge from the people behind the examination—researchers, clinicians, and promoters who commit their endeavors to unwinding the secrets of malignant growth.
Investigate the coordinated efforts and organizations that overcome any barrier between logical development and the lived encounters of those impacted.

In "Voices of Versatility," the individual accounts woven into the texture of logical investigation help us to remember the dauntless human soul and the aggregate strength that arises, notwithstanding quite possibly mankind's most impressive test.

Part 7:

Moral Quandaries and Future Frontiers

In this provocative section, we stand up to the moral predicaments emerging from the advancing scene of malignant growth exploration and treatment. We likewise peer into the future wildernesses, where development and obligation meet, forming the way ahead in the continuous fight against malignant growth.

7.1 The Morals of Disease Research

Look at the moral contemplations inborn in leading malignant growth research, from the utilization of human subjects to the capable treatment of delicate information.

Consider the ethical constraints and difficulties faced by scientists as they continued looking for information and leapfrogged.

7.2 Arising Advancements and Dilemmas

Explore the moral difficulties arising from advancements such as CRISPR and quality altering with regards to malignant growth treatment.

Investigate the almost negligible difference between the potential for noteworthy fixes and the moral ramifications of controlling the human genome.

7.3 Future Wildernesses: Accuracy and Possibilities

Look into the eventual fate of malignant growth treatment, investigating the capability of accurate medication, quality treatments, and other state-of-the art developments.

Think about the moral obligations of offsetting logical advancement with the likely friendly, financial, and moral outcomes.

In thinking about moral problems and future wildernesses, this part energizes reflection on the mindful and evenhanded progression of malignant growth examination and treatment, guaranteeing that logical leaps forward line up with moral standards and cultural prosperity.

Part 8:

Exposing Cell Mysteries

In this part, we set out on an excursion past the limits of disease cells, stripping back the layers of cell secrets to uncover the perplexing dance of life at the tiniest level.

8.1 The Ensemble of Intracellular Communication

Investigate the correspondence networks inside cells, revealing the arrangement of signs that direct cell capabilities.

Analyze the mind-boggling pathways that oversee cell-to-cell correspondence and add to the amicability or dissension inside the cell ensemble.

8.2 Past DNA: Epigenetics and Cell Identity

Expose the job of epigenetics in forming cell character, affecting quality articulation, and cell destiny. Jump into the epigenetic changes that go past the hereditary code, adding intricacy and subtlety to the cell account.

8.3 Organelles: Cell Organs and Their Functions

Look into the particular compartments inside cells, known as organelles, and unwind their imperative jobs in cell processes.

Investigate the unique interaction between organelles, revealing insight into how these cell "organs" contribute to, generally speaking, cell capability.

8.4 From Mitosis to Apoptosis: The Cell Life Cycle

Explore through the periods of the cell life cycle, from cell division (mitosis) to modified cell passing (apoptosis).

Comprehend the finely tuned balance that keeps up with cell homeostasis and the outcomes when this equilibrium is disturbed.

As we expose the secrets inside cells, this section goes beyond the domain of disease to give a far-reaching comprehension of the central cell processes that support life itself.

Part 9:

From Seat to Bedside: Translational Medicine

In this critical section, we navigate the translational scaffold, associating lab disclosures with substantial headways in understanding consideration. Investigate the powerful course of transforming logical experiences into viable applications that can possibly change the scene of malignant growth treatment.

9.1 Benchside Advancements: Divulging Advancement Discoveries

Uncover the most recent weighty revelations rising up out of exploration research facilities, from sub-atomic experiences to promising helpful targets.
Feature the cooperative endeavors of researchers committed to unwinding the intricacies of disease at the benchside.

9.2 Overcoming any Barrier: The Excursion of Translational Research

Explore the difficulties and wins of making an interpretation of lab discoveries into clinical applications.
Investigate the complex idea of translational examination, from preclinical investigations to beginning-stage clinical preliminaries.

9.3 Accuracy Medication Practically speaking, Fitting Medicines to Individuals

- Enlighten the change in outlook towards accuracy medication, where treatment methodologies are redone in view of a singular's special hereditary and atomic profile.
Feature genuine instances of fruitful translational endeavors that have prompted designated treatment with further developed adequacy and diminished incidental effects.

9.4 Difficulties and Amazing Open Doors: Exploring the Translational Landscape

Stand up to the obstacles looked at in the translational excursion, from administrative difficulties to the reconciliation of new advances.
Underline the open doors for joint effort between the scholarly world, industry, and medical service suppliers to speed up the interpretation of logical revelations into substantial patient advantages.

In this part, we span the domains of disclosure and application, investigating how logical information changes into true mediations that hold the possibility of reshaping the scene of malignant growth care

Part 10:

Worldwide Viewpoints on Malignant Growth Difficulties and Collaborations

In this section, expand the focal point to a worldwide scale, looking at the difficulties innate in tending to disease overall and exhibiting cooperative endeavors in the global academic local area.

10.1 The Worldwide Weight of Malignant Growth: A Thorough Overview

Dig into the epidemiological scene, investigating the worldwide prevalence and variety of malignant growth types.

Look at the effect of financial elements, inconsistencies, and social impacts on the rate and results of disease on a worldwide scale.

10.2 Admittance to Malignant Growth Care: Abbreviations and Challenges

Enlighten the variations in admission to malignant growth analysis and treatment across various districts and networks.

Investigate the difficulties in giving fair and reasonable malignant growth care, considering the financial, infrastructural, and social boundaries.

10.3 Cooperative Drives: Joining Powers Against Cancer

Grandstand global joint efforts and drives pointed toward pooling assets, mastery, and information to by and large handle malignant growth.

Feature examples of overcoming the adversity of cooperative examinations, clinical preliminaries, and general wellbeing efforts that have risen above borders.

10.4 Arising Patterns in Worldwide Oncology Research

Investigate arising patterns in worldwide oncology research, from the ascent of global clinical preliminaries to the trading of information and aptitude.

Examine the job of innovation and advancement in spanning holes and cultivating cooperation among analysts, clinicians, and policymakers.

In this part, we explore the perplexing transaction of worldwide elements molding the scene of malignant growth, recognizing the common difficulties while
raising the cooperative undertakings that deal expect a bound together way to deal with disease counteraction, finding, and treatment.

Part 11:

Craftsmanship and Science Impact: The Visual Story of Disease Cells

In this remarkable section, we investigate the crossing point of workmanship and science, delivering the visual portrayals and imaginative translations that convey the magnificence and intricacy of the minute universe of disease cells.

11.1 Minuscule Show-stoppers: Picturing Cell Landscapes

plunge into the universe of tiny imaging methods, exhibiting staggering representations that catch the multifaceted subtleties of malignant growth cells.

Investigate how state-of-the art imaging innovations uncover the excellence concealed inside the cell scene.

11.2 Imaginative Viewpoints: Deciphering the Invisible

Experience imaginative understandings enlivened by the visual style of disease cells, made by craftsmen who team up with researchers to overcome any issues between disciplines.

Consider the cooperative connection between workmanship and science, where inventive articulations add to a more profound comprehension of the cell domain.

11.3 Imparting Intricacy: The Job of Visual Storytelling

Research the effect of visual narrating in science correspondence, utilizing pictures and fine arts to pass complex logical ideas on to different crowds.

Examine how visual stories upgrade public commitment, cultivating a more profound appreciation for the complexities of malignant growth science.

11.4 The Moral Aspects: Craftsmanship, Science, and Representation

Address the moral contemplations encompassing the perception and creative portrayal of malignant growth cells, investigating the harmony between exactness and stylish allure.

Consider how imaginative translations contribute to public discernment and consciousness of malignant growth research.

In this part, we set out on an outwardly rich investigation, where the domains of craftsmanship and science meet to recount a convincing story of the minute world, welcoming perusers to see the value in the excellence and intricacy concealed inside the cell embroidery.

Part 12:

Past the Cells: Effect on Society and Culture

In this broad section, we rise above the logical domain to look at the extensive effect of malignant growth on society and culture. Investigate what this perplexing sickness means for discernments, perspectives, and the more extensive social story.

12.1 Social Viewpoints: Accounts of Trust and Resilience

Explore how social accounts around disease shape public discernments, stressing accounts of trust, versatility, and the human soul.

Investigate social ways to deal with adapting to malignant growth, from conventional mending practices to the impact of cultural mentalities on the patient experience.

12.2 The Language of Disease: Words That Matter

Dive into the phonetic subtleties related to disease, investigating the effect of wording on open talk, shame, and patient encounters.

Examine developing language decisions that add to a more compassionate and engaging discussion around disease.

12.3 Media Portrayals: Forming Public Awareness

Look at the depiction of malignant growth in media, from movies to news inclusion, and its effect on open mindfulness, understanding, and the destigmatization of the sickness.

Dissect both positive and testing portrayals, taking into account their suggestions for molding cultural discernments.

12.4 Social Development and Promotion: Enhancing Voices

Spotlight the job of social developments and promotion in bringing issues to light, destigmatizing disease, and impacting strategy changes.

Investigate how patient backing has turned into a strong force in forming research needs, therapy access, and the more extensive cultural reaction to malignant growth.

This section goes past the logical complexities, welcoming perusers to think about the diverse effect of malignant growth on the structure holding the system together and culture, perceiving its significant impact on language, media, and backing developments.

Part 13:

Unknown Regions: Investigating Rising Frontiers

In this forward-looking part, we adventure into unknown regions, investigating arising wildernesses in disease exploration and treatment. From state-of-the art advancements to creative methodologies, we dig into the potential outcomes that lie ahead.

13.1 Innovative Wonders: The Future Toolbox of Oncology

Study the mechanical headways ready to alter disease exploration and diagnostics, from fluid biopsies to cutting-edge imaging strategies.

Investigate how innovation is extending our capacity to distinguish and grasp disease at prior stages and with more noteworthy accuracy.

13.2 Man-made brainpower in malignant growth: disentangling complexity

Examine the job of man-made reasoning and AI in dissecting huge datasets, recognizing designs, and speeding up disclosures in malignant growth research.

Examine the likely effect of artificial intelligence on customized medication and treatment navigation.

13.3 Hereditary Boondocks: CRISPR and Beyond

Investigate the hereditary boondocks of disease research, including the expected applications and moral contemplations of CRISPR and other quality-altering advances.

Consider how quality treatments might play a groundbreaking role in treating and preventing disease.

13.4 Integrative Methodologies: Comprehensive Disease Care

Analyze comprehensive and integrative ways to deal with disease care, encompassing clinical medicines as well as ways of life, nourishment, and mental prosperity.

Examine how an extensive and patient-driven approach might rethink the eventual fate of disease care.

In Section 13, we look into the future, where the limits of probability are constantly growing. From leading-edge advancements to all-encompassing methodologies, the investigation of unknown domains holds the commitment of reshaping the scene of malignant growth examination and treatment.

Part 14:

Exploring Vulnerability: The Human Experience of Cancer

In this profoundly human section, we explore the close-to-home scenes, vulnerabilities, and groundbreaking minutes that characterize the human experience of malignant growth. From conclusion to survivorship, we dive into the individual stories that enlighten the strength and weakness of those contacted by malignant growth.

14.1 The Snapshot of Conclusion: Exploring Another Reality

Investigate the close-to-home and mental effects of getting a malignant growth conclusion, looking at the prompt difficulties and strategies for dealing with hardship or stress people utilize.
Think about the significant minutes that mark the start of the malignant growth venture and the significance of humane help.

14.2 Treatment Directions: Adjusting Trust and Reality

Explore the assorted directions of disease therapy, from the force of treatments to the nuanced choices around clinical preliminaries and elective methodologies.
Consider the profound cost of treatment and the developing connection among patients and their medical care groups.

14.3 The Scene of Survivorship: Life Past Cancer

Enlighten the encounters of disease survivors, investigating the difficulties and wins they face in the post-treatment stage.
Examine the advancing idea of survivorship and the significance of progressing support and follow-up care.

14.4 Parental figures and friends and family: The Uncelebrated Heroes

Recognize the crucial job of guardians, friends, and family, diving into their encounters, challenges, and the significant effect on the general malignant growth venture.
Think about the elements of care associations and the requirement for all-encompassing help for the two patients and guardians.

Part 14 offers a private investigation of the human elements of malignant growth, revealing insight into the close-to-home shapes, flexibility, and interconnectedness that characterize the significant effect of disease on people and their friends and family.

Part 15:

Past Limits: Worldwide Joint Efforts in Disease Research

In this section, we investigate the force of worldwide joint efforts in propelling malignant growth research, rising above geological limits to pool assets, mastery, and bits of knowledge from different corners of the world.

15.1 The Worldwide Exploration Scene: Organizations Across Continents

Review the present status of global coordinated efforts in disease research, analyzing effective organizations and shared drives.
Investigate how joint efforts empower the trading of information, assets, and viewpoints to speed up progress.

15.2 Multifaceted Points of View: Understanding and Tending to Diversity

Explore the significance of social contemplations in malignant growth research, perceiving the variety of patient populations and their novel necessities.
Examine how worldwide coordinated efforts contribute to a more far-reaching comprehension of disease science and treatment reactions.

15.3 Admittance to Development: Spanning Variations in Disease Care

Look at how worldwide coordinated efforts contribute to further developing access to imaginative medicines, advances, and clinical preliminaries in various areas.
Address the difficulties and valuable open doors in guaranteeing impartial admission to state-of-the art headways.

15.4 Cooperative Exploration Drives: Examples of Overcoming Adversity and Challenges

Grandstand explicit cooperative examination drives that have yielded significant outcomes in the worldwide battle against disease.
Recognize the difficulties inherent in cross-line joint efforts and examine procedures to conquer them

In Part 15, we navigate the interconnected scene of worldwide coordinated efforts in malignant growth research, praising the aggregate endeavors that hold
the possibility to change the direction of disease anticipation, analysis, and treatment around the world.

Part 16:

What was to come Disclosed: Patterns and Prospects in Disease Research

In this forward-looking section, we divulge the eventual fate of malignant growth research, investigating arising patterns, leap forwards, and the potential possibilities that guarantee to shape the scene of oncology in the years to come.

16.1 Cutting-edge Treatments: Advancements on the Horizon
Dive into the pipeline of cutting-edge disease treatments, from novel medication modalities to inventive immunotherapies.
Investigate how headways in remedial methodologies might reclassify the norm of care for different kinds of diseases.

16.2 Biomarker Upheaval: Accuracy, Diagnostics, and Treatment
Look at the advancing job of biomarkers in disease finding, anticipation, and treatment determination.
Talk about the capability of fluid biopsies, sub-atomic profiling, and other biomarker-driven procedures for fitting accurate medication.

16.3 Innovation Incorporation: Large Information, Computer-Based Intelligence, and Beyond
Investigate the combination of large-scale information examination, man-made consciousness, and other cutting-edge innovations in malignant growth research.
Talk about how these innovations might reform information translation, speed up revelations, and customize treatment techniques.

16.4 Patient-Driven Exploration: Engaging the Individual
Examine the shift towards patient-driven research, accentuating shared independent direction, patient-revealed results, and personal satisfaction contemplations.
Investigate how patient association in the research plan and execution adds to additional significant and effective examinations.

In Section 16, we peer into the gem wad of malignant growth research, expecting the patterns and conceivable outcomes that hold the possibility to rethink the fate of oncology, underscoring a patient-focused and mechanically progressed approach.

Part 17:

Moral Outskirts in Malignant Growth Exploration and Treatment

In this basic part, we explore the moral outskirts of malignant growth examination and treatment, tending to complex moral predicaments, contemplations, and the mindful direct of logical request.

17.1 Informed Assent and Independence: Exploring Treatment Choices

Look at the significance of informed consent in disease examination and treatment, regarding people's independence and guaranteeing a reasonable comprehension of expected dangers and advantages. Examine the difficulties in acquiring informed consent, particularly with regards to quickly advancing medicines and trial mediations.

17.2 Value and Access: Moral Contemplations in Asset Allocation

Investigate the moral elements of guaranteeing fair admittance to malignant growth care, treatment choices, and clinical preliminaries.
Address difficulties connected with asset designation, Variations in medical care, and methodologies to advance equity in disease examination and therapy.

17.3 Hereditary Protection and Information Security: Defending Information

Examine the moral ramifications of hereditary data in malignant growth research, accentuating the need to safeguard people's protection and secure delicate information.
Investigate the difficulties and obligations of taking care of hereditary information, especially in the time of genomics and customized medication.

17.4 Mindful Advancement: Adjusting Progress and Risks

Think about the moral obligation of analysts, clinicians, and industry partners to guarantee the dependable turn of events and the execution of imaginative malignant growth treatments.
Talk about systems for assessing the dangers and advantages of new innovations, treatments, and mediations.

In Section 17, we go up against the moral intricacies at the very front of disease exploration and treatment, underscoring the significance of moral standards in directing choices and activities that impact individuals, organizations, and society at large.

Part 18:

The Interconnected Web: Social and Ecological Effects on Cancer

In this interdisciplinary section, we investigate the perplexing associations among social and ecological elements and their effect on malignant growth rate, movement, and results.

18.1 Financial Variations: Effect on Malignant Growth Burden

- Analyze how financial elements, including pay, schooling, and admittance to medical services, contribute to variations in malignant growth hazards, analysis, and results.
Examine systems to address and alleviate financial disparities in disease care and exploration.

18.2 Way of Life and Disease Hazard: Disentangling the Links

Investigate the connections between way of life decisions, like eating routine, active work, and tobacco use, and their effect on disease risk.
Examine general wellbeing interventions and individual ways of behaving that might decrease the general weight of disease.

18.3 Ecological Openings: Recognizing Cancer-Causing Factors

- Research the job of natural openings, including contamination, radiation, and word-related dangers, in adding to disease improvement.
Examine endeavors to recognize and relieve natural variables related to expanded malignant growth risk.

18.4 Social Determinants of Wellbeing: Comprehensive Ways to Deal with Malignant Growth Prevention

Inspect how more extensive social determinants of wellbeing, including schooling, lodging, and local area assets, impact disease results.
Talk about comprehensive ways to deal with malignant growth anticipation that address social determinants and advance wellbeing value.

In Part 18, we unwind the multi-layered trap of social and ecological effects on disease, recognizing the interconnected idea of wellbeing and the significance of taking on exhaustive procedures for malignant growth counteraction and control.

Part 19:

The Force of Avoidance: Techniques and Innovations

In this proactive part, we dive into the domain of disease counteraction, investigating techniques, advancements, and general wellbeing drives pointed toward diminishing the worldwide weight of malignant growth.

19.1 Essential Counteraction: Decreasing Gamble Factors

Look at essential counteraction procedures focusing on modifiable risk factors, like smoking discontinuance, immunization, and way of life intercessions.
Examine the effect of conduct changes on lessening the occurrence of explicit tumors and further developing by and large populace wellbeing.

19.2 Screening and Early Discovery: Disclosing Quiet Threats

Investigate the significance of malignant growth screening and early location endeavors in distinguishing tumors at their most treatable stages.
Examine the difficulties, progressions, and discussions encompassing different screening modalities.

19.3 Immunization as a Preventive Instrument: Past Irresistible Diseases

Research the job of antibodies in forestalling tumors related to irresistible specialists, for example, HPV-related diseases.
Examine continuous endeavors to extend inoculation systems and their expected effect on diminishing malignant growth frequency.

19.4 Accuracy Avoidance: Fitting Ways to Deal with Individuals

Investigate the idea of accuracy, anticipation, and fitting mediations in light of people's hereditary, way of life, and ecological variables.
Talk about how customized avoidance methodologies might add to additional designated and powerful methodologies for diminishing malignant growth risk.

19.5 Local Area Commitment and Training: Engaging Populations

Feature the meaning of local area-based anticipation programs, zeroing in on training, mindfulness, and effort.
Examine fruitful local area commitment drives that enable people and populations to play a functioning role in their wellbeing.

In Part 19, we investigate preventive procedures as well as underline the significance of local area commitment and schooling in engaging people and networks to proactively lessen the effect of malignant growth.

Part 20:

Reflections and Future Horizons

In this finishing up part, we leave on an intelligent excursion, returning to key bits of knowledge, considering the developing scene of disease examination and treatment, and imagining the future skylines that hold the two difficulties and commitments.

20.1 Excursion's End: A Retrospective
Think about the all-encompassing topics, revelations, and stories investigated all through the book, summing up the fundamental learnings.
Consider how the excursion inside the universe of disease cells has extended viewpoints and developed understanding.

20.2 Difficulties and Open Doors: Exploring the Street Ahead
Recognize the tenacious difficulties in the battle against disease, from logical obstacles to moral contemplations and differences in care.
Examine arising open doors and systems to beat impediments, encouraging expectation for progress.

20.3 Voices Representing Things to Come: Forming the upcoming narratives
Enhance the voices of emerging scientists, clinicians, and supporters who address the cutting edge in the area of oncology.
Investigate the developing accounts and goals of those committed to propelling malignant growth research and working on understanding results.

20.4 The Incomplete Story: Embracing Uncertainty
Think about the dynamic and steadily developing nature of the malignant growth account, perceiving that the story is progressing and dependent upon consistent correction.
Embrace the vulnerabilities inborn in chasing after information and progress, recognizing that the mission of understanding malignant growth cells is a getting-through venture.

In Part 20, we bring the story roundtrip, offering an intelligent end that embodies the lavishness of the investigation inside these pages and makes way for the developing story of malignant growth exploration and treatment.

Part 21:

Connecting Disciplines: The Union of Oncology and Technology

In this forward-looking section, we investigate the unique crossing point of oncology and innovation, analyzing how progressions in computerized wellbeing, man-made consciousness, and imaginative advancements are reshaping the scene of malignant growth exploration, conclusion, and treatment.

21.1 Advanced Wellbeing Insurgency: Changing Patient Care
   - Investigate the coordination of advanced wellbeing apparatuses, telemedicine, and remote observing in disease care.
   - Talk about how these advancements upgrade patient commitment, further develop admittance to medical care, and offer customized help all through the disease venture.

21.2 Computerized Reasoning in Oncology: From Diagnostics to Treatment
Research the utilization of man-made brainpower in oncology, including picture examination, prescient demonstration, and treatment improvement.
Examine the capability of man-made intelligence to change demonstrative precision, treatment arrangement, and the advancement of designated treatments.

21.3 Wearable Advancements and Malignant Growth Monitoring
Analyze the job of wearable gadgets in observing disease patients and gathering continuous information on crucial signs, action levels, and treatment reactions.
Examine the potential for wearables to work with early recognition of complexities and work on the general personal satisfaction of disease survivors.

21.4 Developments in Disease Imaging: Past Resolution
Investigate state-of-the-art advancements in disease imaging, from high-goal strategies to atomic imaging advancements.
Examine how best-in-class imaging modalities contribute to early location, exact analysis, and observation of treatment reactions.

21.5 Incorporating Innovation into Disease Exploration and Clinical Trials
Feature how innovation is changing the scene of malignant growth research and clinical preliminaries further developing information assortment, patient enrollment, and preliminary productivity.
Examine the difficulties and amazing open doors in utilizing innovation to speed up the speed of disclosures and advancements in oncology.

In Part 21, we explore the assembly of oncology and innovation, exhibiting how these harmonious progressions are ready to reform the manner in which we comprehend, analyze, and treat malignant growth in the quickly advancing scene of medical services.

Part 22:

The Human Touch in Oncology: Sympathy, Correspondence, and Palliative Care

In this section, we shift the concentration to the fundamental human parts of oncology, investigating the basic job of sympathy, viable correspondence, and palliative consideration in offering comprehensive help to people confronting disease.

22.1 Empathetic Consideration: Sustaining the Patient-Specialist Relationship
Dive into the meaning of empathetic consideration in oncology, accentuating the human association between medical service suppliers and patients.
Examine the effect of compassion, undivided attention, and consistent reassurance on encouraging trust and strength during the malignant growth venture.

22.2 Successful Correspondence: Exploring Troublesome Conversations
Investigate the specialty of compelling correspondence in oncology, especially while passing on troublesome data, talking about treatment choices, and tending to end-of-life care.
Examine methodologies for upgrading relational abilities among medical care experts to guarantee clear and compassionate associations with patients and their families.

22.3 Palliative Consideration: Upgrading the Nature of Life
- Enlighten the job of palliative consideration in supporting patients with disease, overseeing side effects, and improving by and large personal satisfaction.
Examine the combination of palliative consideration into the continuum of disease care, underscoring its advantages in tending to physical, profound, and otherworldly necessities.

22.4 Comprehensive Ways to Deal with Patient Well-Being
Investigate comprehensive ways to deal with patient prosperity, incorporating clinical consideration as well as mental, social, and otherworldly help.
Examine the significance of multidisciplinary groups in tending to the different requirements of patients and elevating an extensive way to deal with disease care.

22.5 Parental Figure Backing: Perceiving and Tending to Their Needs
Recognize the critical role of guardians in the disease venture and investigate methodologies to give them the help, assets, and acknowledgment they need.
Talk about the difficulties looked at through parental figures and drives pointed toward advancing their prosperity.

In Part 22, we stress the human touch in oncology, perceiving that past the logical and mechanical progressions, empathetic consideration, compelling correspondence, and an emphasis on general prosperity are necessary to offering exhaustive help to people impacted by disease.

Part 23:

Worldwide Backing and Strategy: Molding the Oncology Landscape

In this section, we dive into the domain of worldwide promotion and strategy, investigating how aggregate endeavors, informed arrangements, and backing drives assume a critical role in forming the scene of oncology on an overall scale.

23.1 Pushing for Patient Privileges: Engaging Voices

Investigate the role of patient backing in molding arrangements, advancing mindfulness, and enabling people impacted by malignant growth.

feature effective support crusades that have added to strategy changes and worked on the patient experience.

23.2 Strategy Structures in Malignant Growth Control: Exploring Challenges

Analyze existing arrangements for malignant growth control at the public and worldwide levels. Examine difficulties in arrangement execution, holes in medical services frameworks, and expected procedures for defeating boundaries to compelling disease control.

23.3 Worldwide Wellbeing Tact: Coordinated efforts for Disease Control

Investigate the crossing point of worldwide wellbeing tactics and disease control, accentuating the significance of global coordinated efforts, associations, and conciliatory endeavors.

Talk about examples of overcoming adversity and moves to encourage worldwide participation to address the intricacies of disease anticipation, treatment, and examination.

23.4 Wellbeing Financial Matters and Access: Adjusting Cost and Care

Examine the monetary contemplations in disease care, resolving issues of moderateness, admittance to therapies, and the financial weight of malignant growth on people and medical service frameworks. Examine strategy approaches pointed toward adjusting the expense adequacy of mediations with the requirement for fair admission to top-notch malignant growth care.

23.5 Future Headings in Oncology Strategy: A Call to Action

Think about future headings and arising needs in oncology strategy, including the coordination of new advances, tending to wellbeing differences, and encouraging development.

Propose a source of inspiration for policymakers, medical services experts, backers, and people to team up to mold a more successful and fair oncology scene.

In Section 23, we investigate the powerful job of promotion and strategy in the worldwide battle against malignant growth, perceiving that educated approaches and aggregate backing endeavors are pivotal for making a system that upholds viable disease control, admittance to mind, and progressions in oncology research.

Part 24:

The Strength of the Human Soul: Accounts of Win and Hope

In this helpful part, we dive into accounts of win and trust, commending the versatility of people who have confronted malignant growth with mental fortitude, assurance, and a soul that rises above the difficulties of the sickness.

24.1 Individual Accounts: Voices of Triumph

Share individual accounts of people who have prevailed over disease, featuring their excursions, difficulties, and snapshots of strength.
Feature different stories that mirror the strength and variety of the human soul, even with difficulty.

24.2 Advancements in Steady Consideration: Improving the Patient Experience

Investigate developments in strong consideration that mean to upgrade the general patient experience during and after disease treatment.
Examine drives, projects, and mediations that focus on the close-to-home, mental, and social prosperity of people impacted by disease.

24.3 Patient-Driven Drives: Enabling the Community

Feature drives driven by patients and survivors that add to mindfulness, backing, and backing inside the malignant growth local area
Examine the effect of patient-driven developments on impacting research needs, strategy changes, cultivating a sense of local area, and strengthening

24.4 Coordinating Craftsmanship and Wellbeing: Imaginative Articulations in Healing

Investigate the role of imaginative and innovative articulations in advancing healing, flexibility, and prosperity among people impacted by malignant growth.
Talk about drives that incorporate craftsmanship, music, and different types of inventive articulation into malignant growth care to improve the general recuperating experience.

24.5 A Brief Look into What's to Come: Trust on the Horizon

Give a brief look into future prospects and arising patterns that may expect people to confront disease.
Examine how progressing headways, steady organizations, and the aggregate versatility of the human soul add to a more promising time to come in the battle against disease.

In Part 24, we commend the dauntless soul of the people who have explored the difficult territory of disease, accentuating that accounts of win and strongly expect rouse, as well as adding to the aggregate strength of the worldwide local area impacted by malignant growth.

Part 25:

Reflections on the Excursion: An Embroidery of Understanding

In this intelligent part, we delay to wind around together the strings of understanding developed all through this investigation of malignant growth cells, exploration, treatment, and the human experience.

25.1 Illustrations Learned: Experiences from the Infinitesimal Realm

Think about key examples gained from the tiny investigation of malignant growth cells, taking into account the intricacies, variations, and weaknesses uncovered.

25.2 The Steadily Changing Scene of Oncology

Mull over the powerful idea of the oncology scene, perceiving how logical headways, mechanical developments, and cultural impacts ceaselessly reshape the account.

25.3 Unanswered Inquiries and Frontiers

Recognize the constant secrets and unanswered inquiries in malignant growth research, underscoring the wildernesses that coax investigation and disclosure.

25.4 The Woven Artwork of the Joint Aim: Voices Unite

Praise the cooperative endeavors of researchers, medical services experts, backers, and people impacted by malignant growth, perceiving the force of aggregate voices in propelling comprehension and care.

25.5 The Human Side of Malignant Growth: A Call for Compassion

Stress the significance of sympathy, powerful correspondence, and steady consideration on the human side of disease, highlighting the meaning of a comprehensive methodology.

25.6 The Future Unfurling: Seeds of Hope

Sow seeds of expectation for the future, imagining a scene where research leaps forward, mechanical developments, and sympathetic consideration keep on making ready for progress.

In Section 25, we step back to see the value in the complexities of the excursion, perceiving that understanding disease isn't just about disentangling its atomic secrets yet additionally embracing human stories, cooperative endeavors, and the steadily advancing embroidered artwork that characterizes the continuous journey for information and progress in the domain of oncology.

Index:

Assets and Further Reading

In this far-reaching reference section, perusers will find an organized rundown of assets and proposed readings to dive further into different parts of disease research, treatment, patient help, and promotion. The supplement fills in as a significant aide for those looking for extra data, references, and points of view on the complex scene of malignant growth.

A.1 Logical Diaries and Publications

A gathering of legitimate logical diaries and distributions in the area of oncology, furnishing perusers with admittance to the most recent examination, surveys, and leap forwards.

A.2 Patient Help Organizations

A rundown of perceived patient help associations offering data, assets, and local area associations for people and families impacted by malignant growth

A.3 Suggested Books for Additional Reading

A determination of books covering a scope of points connected with malignant growth, including journals, logical investigations, and stories that give bits of knowledge into the human experience of the illness.

A.4: Instructive Sites and Online Platforms

A combination of instructive sites and online stages committed to disease training, mindfulness, and giving solid data to patients, guardians, and the overall population.

A.5 Exploration Organizations and Centers

A list of famous examination foundations and malignant growth places around the world where state-of-the art research, clinical preliminaries, and progressions in disease treatment are led

A.6 Strategy and Backing Resources

Assets zeroing in on malignant growth backing, strategy drives, and associations pursuing molding approaches for disease avoidance, treatment, and backing

A.7 Glossary of Terms

A glossary giving definitions to key terms and wording utilized all through the book, guaranteeing clarity and understanding for perusers.

A.8 Acknowledgments

A segment offering thanks to people, associations, and benefactors who played a critical role in the creation and improvement of the book.

This far-reaching index means to be a significant sidekick, directing perusers to investigate further, draw in respectable assets, and extend how they might interpret the different features of malignant growth.